Fertility & Infertility

The Unexpected Explained

Introduction

This book contains complete details of fertility and infertility.

The term "infertility" is used to describe the inability of a woman or a man to conceive a child or the inability of a woman to carry a pregnancy to term.

Infertility is defined clinically in men and women who do not achieve a pregnancy after one year of unprotected sex. In women older than 35 years, this period is reduced to 6 months to indicate that in this age group an earlier evaluation is advised, since fertility is reduced with age.

Many different diseases and other factors can contribute to the development of fertility problems. A particular case may have a single cause of infertility, several or — in some cases — no identifiable cause.

Different scientists supported by the Institute are conducting research to identify both the causes of infertility and new treatments that could help men and women achieve a pregnancy and women to carry a pregnancy to term.

I hope you enjoy it!

Chapter 1: Fertility & Infertility: General

Fertility is the ability you have to conceive a child. This occurs when the ovum fuses with a sperm while it is in one of the fallopian tubes. In most cases, fertility occurs to almost all men and women, but there are cases in which they are infertile, that is, they cannot have children following traditional methods. There are, however, ways of conceiving alternatives.

The fertility of women is closely related to their age: from 40 years, the percentage of infertility reaches 50%, which finally ends with menopause. Men, on the other hand, have a higher rate of fertility, although age also affects their fertility.

In general, leading a healthy life usually implies good levels of fertility.

➤ It is the ability to have children

➤ Women are fertile around thirty-five years of their life, between puberty and menopause (from the first menstruation until the last) and at this stage of their life they are fertile only on certain days each month, when the mature ovum comes out of the ovary

➤ The man is fertile most of his life, which means that the man can embarrass the woman in any sexual relation that it has, if it coincides with the fertile days of her. Sperm production begins to decrease after the fifth decade of men's lives.

What Is Infertility?

Infertility is the inability of both men and women, of having children. A couple is considered infertile, when after a year of frequent, unprotected sex, they can not conceive. If you want to have a child, both should go to the doctor, because the cause may be in the man, or in the woman or both.

What Are The Main Causes Of Female Infertility?

The main causes of female infertility are difficulties in ovulation (not ovulating or not frequent in ovulation), occlusion of uterine tubas or fallopian tubes, endometriosis, among others. The lack of ovulation can be due to problems in the ovaries, such as hormonal imbalance, some chronic disease and poor nutrition, and tubal problems are usually due to sexually transmitted infections.

Can Man Be Infertile?

Yes, there are several causes that can cause infertility in man, the most common being the following:

> Problems in the testes sexually transmitted infections sequelae of mumps (mumps) blows in the testicles

> Genetic problems

> Retrograde ejaculation, decreased semen quality

What Can Be The Factors That Cause The Semen Quality To Be Decreased?

> Use of drugs (alcohol, marijuana, cocaine)

> Infections or diseases.

> Chromosomal abnormalities.

> Use of herbicides and pesticides, without taking protective measures.

> Prolonged exposure to x-rays, or in workplaces with high temperatures, for example, factories, furnaces, boilers.

How Can You Know When Is The Fertile Period?

Ovulation is what marks the fertile period of each woman and it is difficult to know exactly when it happens, however, you can have a fairly approximate idea if you follow the following steps:

> The fertile days of a woman depend on the length of her menstrual cycle, which can vary from 26 to 34 days.

> The woman must mark on a calendar for between eight and twelve months, the days of her menstruation, that is, from the first day of her period to the last.

> Once indicated at least eight cycles, count how many days pass from the first day of the rule until the day before the next bleeding.

> If the cycles are regular, that is, they always last the same number of days, be it 24, 27, 28 or 30 days, you can know that you have regular cycles and that it is feasible to use this method.

> If the cycles do not always last the same, that is, a month lasts 26, another 28 and another 30 days, it means that the final document has an irregular cycle, so it is very difficult to identify the day of ovulation and, therefore, so much, the fertile days.

> If you have a regular cycle you can identify the possible day of ovulation by subtracting 14 days from the date that the next rule is supposed to come.

> The fertile days of the month are the five days before and five days after the day of ovulation

How Long Is The Fertile Period?

About ten days: five before and five after the day that ovulation is expected, because you have to take into account the life cycle of an egg that is about 24 hours and that of a sperm that is 72, and while both If they are alive and found, pregnancy may occur.

It can happen that they have sex two or three days before the probable date of ovulation, but since the sperm remain alive in the tubes for up to three days, it is possible that the sperm can fertilize the egg on the day of its release.

Chapter 2: Unexplained Infertility

Fertility is the ability you have to conceive a child. This occurs when the ovum fuses with a sperm while it is in one of the fallopian tubes. In most cases, fertility occurs to almost all men and women, but there are cases in which they are infertile, that is, they cannot have children following traditional methods. There are, however, ways of conceiving alternatives.

"Why I Can Not Have A Baby?"

For people diagnosed with unexplained infertility, the journey of parenting can be particularly difficult. The San Diego Fertility Center recognizes that not understanding why you are unable to conceive is a unique and frustrating experience. Couples are left with unanswered questions about the cause of their inability to get pregnant, and what, in any case, can be done to treat it.

Our team of fertility specialists works with individuals and couples looking to build their family when a definitive fertility problem can be identified. Unexplained infertility does not have to mean giving up your dream of starting a family. In fact, many of our patients are able to succeed a baby after trying a single treatment to help increase the likelihood of conception.

What Is Unexplained Infertility?

For 20 to 30 percent of couples (and up to 80 percent of women around age 40), fertility testing will lead to a diagnosis of "unexplained infertility. "This diagnosis is given after a Complete diagnostic study does not reveal a specific cause for the woman's inability to conceive. The diagnosis implies that there is a problem, but doctors cannot find a definitive explanation or prescribe an exact treatment.

What Are The Causes Of Unexplained Infertility?

Age is one of the most common causes of unexplained infertility. Women 35 years of age or older have a higher incidence of this diagnosis, and women older than 38 years have a higher incidence. Women older than 40 who are still ovulating regularly, unexplained infertility is probably due to ovum quality problems that are not easily determined.

Due to the hundreds of molecular and biochemical processes that must happen perfectly in order for a pregnancy to occur, unexplained infertility is probably caused by a number of factors. Standard fertility tests focus on obvious issues such as irregularities in ovulation and abnormal sperm counts.

How Is Unexplained Infertility Diagnosed?

A woman is diagnosed with unexplained infertility if she is not successful in pregnancy and all standard fertility tests for her and her partner are normal. In such cases, this means that the following is present:

> - The physical exam shows no signs of abnormalities in the uterus, Fallopian tubes or ovaries
> - All ovarian reserve tests show normal levels of egg supply.
> - Hysterosalpingography (HSG or) shows normal tubes of the uterine cavity and fallopian tubes.
> - The semen analysis of the man shows adequate amounts of healthy sperm.
> - The ovulation activity of the woman is normal, or any ovulation disorder (such as polycystic ovarian syndrome) have been successfully treated.
> - All blood tests of both sexes show normal results.

Your doctor will study all test results before providing a diagnosis of unexplained infertility.

Can You Treat Unexplained Infertility?

There are different Fertility Centers committed to giving each couple the best chance of having a baby by using cutting-edge technologies to help improve pregnancy outcomes. Some ways we treat unexplained infertility include:

> ➢ In Vitro Fertilization (IVF) - IVF has high success rates for women with unexplained infertility who have normal ovarian reserve tests.

> ➢ Clomid and intrauterine insemination (IAI) - Clomid (clomiphene citrate) is a pill used to treat ovulation problems that is used to greatly improve fertility rates especially during an IAI cycle.

> ➢ Letrozole or Femara - this oral medication is sometimes used to stimulate the development of multiple follicles during the treatment of infertility.

> ➢ Injections of hormones FSH and IAI - these injectable drugs stimulate the development of multiple follicles during the treatment of infertility and is generally used in conjunction with IAI.

> ➢ Clomid and sexual intercourse - Clomid can be used with scheduled intercourse as a low-level fertility treatment.

Chapter 3: What Is Infertility?

Being a parent is not easy. The children test us constantly: sometimes they get the best out of you but sometimes the worst too. It is difficult to control, but it is worth it. Studies show that anger and physical punishment to children cause their resentment and feel bad about themselves.

On the contrary, the mixture of communication with discipline and affection teaches them to behave and develop in a healthy and independent way. They feel that they are heard and valued. These are some of the principles of positive parenting, a methodology developed in 1920 by Alfred Adler and Rudolf Dreikurs. Teach children to become responsible and respectful people.

The little ones in the house behave badly, and the parents have to face it. Parents can react with anger, shouting, bad humor and punishments or just the opposite: calm, understanding, communication to achieve positive discipline. This concept does not imply punishment, but to teach your child to behave. The whipping or cheeks can work in the short term, but the child does not correct his attitude because you have motivated him to control himself but for fear of a repeat of the slap.

Positive discipline does not mean being excessively strict nor permissive. It is about setting limits so that they learn to be self-disciplined. Let them get used to putting limits on themselves.

In addition, they provide security and provide a strong bond with the children, provided that they are established with love, affection and empathy, from understanding, so they can internalize and think for themselves. Saying "no" often weakens the relationship.

Positive Parenting: Setting Limits To Achieve Self-Discipline

What limits to put?

> First, those who promote your safety and theirs. Those are not negotiable. Although it is likely to change as your child grows. Make sure they are chords for your age. Others will be given by the needs of the child (sleep, food...). In short, it is about responding to the child's development needs.

> Avoid unnecessary limits. The ones that you put, always with affection to strengthen the relationship. Each person is different, so each one may need different rules.

> Children raised with attachment become less angry and develop a sense of responsibility earlier. As they grow up, they show more cooperation with their parents; they get along better with their classmates, they learn faster in school, their self-esteem is greater, and they resist stressing better. Without that cordiality the child does not collaborate but is rebellious.

Children Of An Authoritarian Education

Sometimes it can be difficult for parents to control themselves, but authoritarian paternity harms the emotional development of children. They do not learn to self-regulate, but they are reluctant to take responsibility. They reject that limit because they feel bad if they are told things in a bad way and without attachment. And they respond to him out of fear, because they feel intimidated. They obey but do not think for themselves. Moreover, adults are not going to question the authority when they should. It is shown that authoritatively raised children are more prone to anger, depression and rebellion. A too demanding upbringing deteriorates the relationship between parents and children.

Children Of Permissive Parents

By not provoking a tantrum or making their children unhappy, some parents do not set limits and educate the children in permissiveness. And this has a negative effect because they do not learn to tolerate frustration, disappointment and sadness. Getting away with it can always hinder the creation of friendships, as they become egocentric.

Objective: To Help Your Child Feel Good And To Learn To Function Alone

Positive discipline or parenting guides children by creating a close bond. In this way, they always try to please the parents. With punishments, they feel angry and in the long run their behavior does not improve. And it encourages them to be more influenced by friends or colleagues than by their parents.

> ➢ If you apply anger, they will copy that model themselves. Try to understand them to set limits. Discuss and discuss your point of view and yours, about the consequence of your actions. Make it feel like a learning experience.

> ➢ To strengthen that relationship, try to speak positively, to say "yes" instead of "no," even when imposing a limit. Change your language and "eat" your anger through self-control. They change us for the better; they can draw our most positive side. For them we are able to give everything. Any conflict or problem is solved better from tranquility and calm. That is sometimes not easy but breathes deeply. Do not make a decision in hot, wait a while. Find a constructive reaction.

A good communication, i.e. listening and speaking (avoiding interrupt) is vital in your relationship with your child, even if it is sometimes complicated. Acquire that habit by reserving a time for it daily. And if you cannot when they ask for it, simply tell them that now it cannot be, but later. So they know that you are always there to help them with any problem.

Chapter 4: How To Deal With Infertility?

First of all it is necessary to look for the resources of medicine, and then...

In the first place it is necessary to look for the resources of medicine. There are many causes that can cause infertility. For the man it can be, for example, a hormonal problem: low level of testosterone or prolactin; This can be detected through exams in a consultation with an endocrinologist.

Also the Varicocele can cause infertility in man; as well as the low number of sperm (hypospermia); An exam ordered by the urologist can detect the counting, quality and motor skills of them.

In relation to women, you should consult a gynecologist and endocrinologist; Any gland with an unbalanced function in women can lead to infertility. Thus, the ovaries, the adrenal, thyroid, pituitary, etc., need to be examined.

In addition to that, there may be uterine problems such as fibroids, polyps, endometriosis, which can be resolved in many cases with surgery. Also, the congenital malformations that can impede fertility.

Some doctors also point to the psychological factor of the woman, sometimes the anxiety of wanting to get pregnant can hinder pregnancy; there are many cases of women who manage to get pregnant after adopting a child... For this type of problem, psychological support is recommended.

The Billings method can help a woman get pregnant; If you learn well how to detect the days of fertility, when a uterine mucus appears, you will be more likely to get pregnant if you have sex in those days. There are simple books that teach the method.

The Catholic Church understands that the generation of a child must happen only through the action of the parents; that is why it does not accept "in vitro" fertilization (baby test tube).

The Catechism of the Church explains that: " The techniques that cause a dissociation of kinship, by the intervention of a person outside the couple (donor of sperm or egg, belly rent), are seriously dishonest. These techniques (heterologous artificial insemination and fecundation) undermine the child's right to be born of a father and mother known to him and linked by marriage. They betray the exclusive right to become father and mother only through the other "(Congregation for the Doctrine of the Faith, Instruction Donum Vitae, 2.1).

Practiced among the couple, these techniques (artificial insemination and fertilization homologous) are perhaps less clear to an immediate trial, but still cause moral problems. Dissociate the sexual act of the procreative act.

The fundamental act of the existence of the children is no longer an act by which two people donate one to the other, but an act that " remits the life and identity of the embryo to the power of the doctors and biologists, and establishes a mastery of the technique over the origin and destiny of the human person. Such a relationship of ownership is in itself contrary to the dignity and equality that should be common to both parents and children "(CDF, Instrument DV, II, 741.5).

"Procreation is morally deprived of its perfection when it is not wanted as a result of the conjugal act, that is, of the specific gesture of union of the spouses... Only respect for the link that exists between the meanings of the conjugal act and respect for unity of the human being allows a procreation according to the dignity of the person "

But the Church accepts medical treatments so that the man or woman can reach fertility.

"Research that tends to diminish human sterility must be stimulated, under the condition of being placed at the service of the human person, of their inalienable rights, of their true and integral good, in accordance with the project and will of God".

But the fact that the couple cannot have children does not mean that their marriage has lost its meaning.

The Church says that: "Spouses to whom God has not granted to have children can lead a conjugal life full of meaning, humanly and Christianly. Their marriage can radiate a fecundity of charity, welcome and sacrifice "(§1654).

And the couple can live their sex life normally, because if there is no procreative aspect in the couple, there is at least the unitive one.

The Church knows that "great is the suffering of the spouses who discover themselves sterile" (§2374).

For those couples, the Church recommends adoption and says that " the Gospel teaches that physical sterility is not an absolute evil. The spouses who, having exhausted the legitimate resources of medicine, suffer from sterility, must associate themselves with the Cross of the Lord, the source of all spiritual fruitfulness. They can manifest their generosity by adopting abandoned children or performing self-sacrificing services for the benefit of others "(§2379).

Above all, the Christian couple must face infertility in the faith; "We know that in all things God intervenes for the good of those who love him " (Rm 8,28) and "Give thanks in all circumstances" (1 Thesis 5:18).

The couple should not question God "why" not to have children, but surrender in their divine hands to the faith, although this is difficult.

The Bible gives us examples of sterile women who prayed to God and managed to get pregnant; So it was with the mother of Samuel and Samson.

Jesus commanded: "Ask and you will receive, seek and you will find, play and it will be opened to you". Therefore, in faith, the Christian couple must ask for the son so desired to God, and make like the holy women of the Bible: offer that child to God, even before being conceived.

The prayers can be varied: in front of the Most Holy, the Rosary to the Virgin, in the Eucharistic communion, in the novenas and litanies, in short, with all the means you can and know how to pray.

If even with all this, the son did not come, "may the will of God be done", certainly He has some design that we do not know, but that faith is a guarantor for the good of the couple.

It is the hour of faith, but it is also the hour of consolation, only this faith can give, in fact, to the couple peace and happiness.

Chapter 5: Signs Of Infertility In Men And Women

Knowing the signs of infertility in men and women that can attract attention and that may suggest that there is a problem in a couple to achieve pregnancy is something that many couples claim to know and that we will try to explain in this article. It is not always easy to recognize which signs of infertility can alert us, but it is important to know them to know when to go to a specialist in reproductive medicine.

When To Go To A Reproduction Clinic

The sign of classic infertility that should make a couple go to an assisted reproduction clinic is the time of pregnancy search. If a couple has been having unprotected sex for a year without having reached gestation, it is convenient to go to an assisted reproduction clinic to perform a sterility study. However, depending on the characteristics of the couple, these times can be modified. For example, if the woman is over 40 years old it might be advisable not to wait more than 6 months. However, in very young patients can be rushed up to a year and a half before going to consultation in the reproduction clinic.

Other Signs Of Infertility In Men And Women

As we have said, gestation search time is the most important warning sign that a couple can have. However, there may be other signs of infertility that can attract attention in both men and women. In the case of women, we can highlight:

➢ **Irregular rules:** the presence of irregular rules in a woman may suggest the existence of ovulatory problems that hinder the arrival of pregnancy

➢ **Previous abdominal surgeries:** the existence of inflammatory processes in the abdomen and, above all, surgeries, can be a risk factor for the existence of reproductive problems due to possible injuries and adhesions in the fallopian tubes.

> **History of infection in the internal genital tract**. Tubal and ovarian infections are an important risk factor for reproductive problems

> **History of endometriosis:** if the patient knows that she has an endometriosis, this can be a risk factor for having problems to get pregnant

> **Previous treatments** of chemo and / or radiotherapy: these treatments can injure the ovaries and cause problems to get a pregnancy

In the case of the male we can take into account the following signs:

> **Painful or not in the testicles:** these may be signs of problems in the testicles that affect the production of sperm

> **Previous history of lack of descent** of the testicles to the scrotal sac. Since the testicle must work at a lower temperature than the rest of the body, this lack of descent can cause sperm production to decrease

> **Previous history of infections** and traumatisms in the testicle: these infections and traumatisms can leave residual lesions that hinder the arrival of pregnancy

> **History of mumps contracted** during puberty. If this disease is contracted during the pubertal development of the testicle, it can cause lesions in it that make it difficult for the pregnancy to arrive

> **I work in very hot or long seated environments** or with environmental toxins for the testicle such as inks, tails, etc. All these jobs can cause lesions to the testicle that decrease the production of sperm

> **Previous treatments of chemo and / or radiotherapy**: these treatments can also injure the testicles and cause problems to get a pregnancy

As we can see, there is an important variety of signs of infertility in both men and women. However, as it is not always easy to recognize which sign may be relevant and which is not, consult any specialist in assisted reproduction. This can advise you on possible problems that may or may not be having.

Chapter 6: Factors That Can Affect Your Fertility

Could I have a fertility problem?

If you are under 35 and have been trying to get pregnant for less than a year (or less than six months if you are over 35), there is still no reason to worry. If you want to be sure you are doing everything possible to increase your chances of getting pregnant, read our articles on how to detect ovulation and use our ovulation calculator and guide on vaginal discharge, to know when you are most fertile.

If you are under 35 and have had frequent unprotected sex for more than a year (or for at least six months, if you are over 35 years old.), and you have not managed to conceive, there are quite a few chances that you or your partner have a complication that is interfering with the conception, but only a doctor can diagnose with certainty the existence of a fertility problem.

It is estimated that one in ten couples has problems conceiving. If you are one of them, this does not mean that you will never have children. Many couples who try to have children will manage to have them by their own means — 50 percent will do so during the first year — but many others will need medical intervention to conceive.

What factors are linked to women's fertility problems?

If you have any of the following complications, tell the doctor. Maybe there is something that can be corrected by a treatment or a change in daily habits, and it is better to do it as soon as possible, instead of spending six months or a year trying to conceive naturally.

Background Of:

➢ Endometriosis
➢ Uterine fibroids

- Polycystic ovary syndrome
- Pelvic inflammatory disease
- Fallopian tube obstruction due to infection or previous surgery
- Sexually transmitted infections such as chlamydia or gonorrhea
- Irregular or painful periods
- Excessive facial or body hair
- Pelvic or abdominal surgery
- Exposure to DES in utero (DES is a drug that was given to pregnant women to prevent spontaneous abortions between 1941 and 1971.)
- **A chronic disease such as diabetes, cancer or a disease of the thyroid gland Or if you currently:** smoke, or find yourself 25 percent below or above the appropriate weight for you.

What factors are linked to man's fertility problems?

As in the previous case, it is best to consult your doctor if you have any of the following complications, to study the possibility of a treatment or a change of habits.

Background Of:

- Mumps virus infection after puberty
- Chronic disease such as diabetes, cancer or a condition of the thyroid gland
- One or both testes have not descended (cryptorchidism)
- Tumors, cysts, cancer or varicoceles in the testicles

Or If Currently:

- Take medications such as steroids or antidepressants
- You smoke tobacco or marijuana
- Do you use the Jacuzzi or sauna regularly

➤ You make frequent long bicycle trips

What should I do if I suspect there may be a problem?

Tell your doctor or gynecologist. Do not hesitate to consult any concern or fear you have, regardless of how long you have been trying to get pregnant.

Surely the doctor can answer your questions or, if necessary, advise you to consult a fertility specialist to make a diagnosis.

Chapter 7: Difference Between Infertility & Sterility

Although many times these two terms are used as synonyms, because they refer to the impossibility of having a baby, in reality they are not. We tell you what differences there are between infertility and sterility.

It is not uncommon to hear the terms sterility and infertility in today's society. But we do not always listen to them with good use of their definition. For that reason, from Being Parents, we wanted to make the difference and treat both terms separately with the intention of explaining what sterility is and what is infertility.

The sterility is the inability to achieve pregnancy. In general terms, a couple is considered sterile when, after a year of sexual intercourse without contraceptive methods, pregnancy is not achieved. We can differentiate between:

- **Primary sterility**: if the couple has never managed to have a child.
- **Secondary sterility**: if after having had children a new pregnancy is not achieved.

Sometimes, sterility occurs from external causes. And in that list, the stress, the rhythm of life of the couple, their habits or their diet have a lot to say.

Infertility

On the other hand, there is talk of infertility when a woman has achieved one or more pregnancies, but they have not reached term or the death of the baby has occurred hours after delivery. We can distinguish between:

- **Primary infertility:** the woman becomes pregnant, but the pregnancy does not come to term or the baby dies shortly after birth.

> ➢ **Secondary infertility:** the couple has a healthy baby, after a normal pregnancy and delivery. When they go back to look for a baby, even if they get pregnant, it does not get to term.

How Long Does It Take To Get Pregnant?

96 percent of couples who have unprotected sex achieve pregnancy around 12 months of trying. Therefore, specialists recommend waiting at least all that time before undergoing a fertility study.

The problems to get pregnant are related to many factors. One of the most important is the age of the woman, since at 35 the monthly possibility of becoming pregnant is 10%, while at 40 it is only 5%. This does not mean that a woman over 35 can not have more children, but will need more time to get it.

Not only that. Another factor that influences and not little in that a pregnancy is achieved is the stress that both parties of the couple or only one have. It is proven that the greater the stress, the lower the chances of getting a pregnancy. The same happens when there are unhealthy habits in men or women or both. For this type of habits is understood smoking, sedentary lifestyle and obviously a bad diet.

Therefore, when you want to have a baby, it is important to take care of what we eat and what we drink, not abusing alcohol and of course not smoking. Otherwise, we will be increasing the chances of failure in the baby project.

Chapter 8: Fertility Tests

Fertility tests are the best way to know if you are infertile and can help you find the cause. If you have been looking for a pregnancy for more than 1 year, see a doctor.

How Can I Know If I Am Infertile?

It can be difficult to determine if you are really infertile. Often there are no signs of infertility, except for the inability to achieve or maintain a pregnancy. The only way to know for sure is to see a doctor and get tested for infertility.

When Should I See A Doctor To Do The Infertility Tests?

It is normal to take up to a year to achieve a pregnancy. If you have tried for more than 1 year and you have not had any luck, it is a good idea to consult a doctor about the possibility of testing for infertility.

Some health problems can make it harder to achieve a pregnancy. Do not wait a year to talk to the doctor if you or your partner have any of these antecedents:

- Ectopic pregnancy
- Irregular menstrual periods
- Pelvic inflammatory disease
- Repeated miscarriages
- Problems of the thyroid gland
- Cystic fibrosis
- Injuries or trauma to the scrotum or testicles
- Difficulty having an erection
- Ejaculation problems

Some doctors recommend that women over 35 be tested for infertility after 6 months of trying to get pregnant.

Your GP or gynecologist can perform infertility tests or refer you to a fertility specialist. At the local Planned Parenthood health center, they can also help you find where to perform fertility tests in your area.

What Happens During A Fertility Test?

Tests for infertility detection usually begin with a nurse or doctor who asks you about your medical history and performs a physical exam. It may take several months for your doctor to detect what is causing your fertility problems, so do not be discouraged if you do not get an immediate response.

Fertility Tests For Ovules, Uterus, Fallopian Tubes:

The doctor will perform a pelvic exam. You can also use ultrasound to see your ovaries and uterus, and indicate a blood test to monitor your hormones. Sometimes it is necessary to follow your ovulation pattern by checking the cervical mucus, taking the temperature or using ovulation tests at home.

Usually, if the answer is not found in the first exams, then other tests and procedures are performed. A special test called "hysterosalpingogram" is done to see if the fallopian tubes are open. The doctor places a dye in the uterus and then observes with X-ray equipment how the dye travels through the uterus and fallopian tubes.

In some cases, infertility tests may include minor surgeries to explore inside your body. The doctor will use special tools to check the fallopian tubes, ovaries, and uterus to see if there are problems.

Sperm And Semen Fertility Tests:

This class of fertility tests usually includes a physical exam and a semen analysis. The semen is analyzed to know the following:

> ➢ Sperm count (how many sperm are in your semen)

- ➢ How fast your sperm move
- ➢ The size, shape and quality of your sperm
- ➢ The amount of seminal fluid

You can also have a blood test to find out if there is a hormonal problem that makes it difficult for you to cause a pregnancy.

How Is Infertility Treated?

There are several types of infertility treatments. The best options for you depend on the cause of your fertility problems. Sometimes only one of the people in the couple needs treatment; others, both have to use a combination of treatments.

The treatment of infertility can include a combination of lifestyle changes, medications, hormonal therapy and surgical procedures. If there is a problem with sperm or eggs, sperm or donor eggs may be used. Two of the most common fertility treatments are intrauterine insemination and in vitro fertilization (IVF). Get more information about fertility treatments.

The treatment of infertility usually begins with consultation with a doctor who specializes in pregnancy and infertility. Your GP or your gynecologist can refer you to a fertility specialist. It is also possible to get fertility treatments or help finding a fertility specialist in your area at the local Planned Parenthood health center.

Conclusion

A woman is fertile since she has her first period, but her capacity diminishes with age. In the case of men, there is also a gradual decrease, although later and less pronounced.

For many reasons, women decide to have their children later and later. So, every day is more normal to face difficulties at that time. If a few years ago, the Assisted Reproduction Techniques were for a few, today these are a usual practice.

What is the difference between sterility and infertility?

Infertility can easily be as the inability to conceive a pregnancy. It can be of feminine or masculine origin. The sterile couple is considered when after a year of unprotected sexual intercourse pregnancies is not achieved. The concept of sterility must be distinguished from that of infertility. Primary sterility is called that in which there have never been pregnancies and secondary sterility refers to the situation in which there have been previous pregnancies and then the impossibility of new pregnancies.

In infertility, women get pregnancies, but pregnancy ends in abortion. In short, sterility is when you are not able to get pregnant, and infertility when in spite of getting the pregnancy, it is not carried to term. It should be noted that in the Anglo-Saxon countries, the term "infertility" includes both concepts, which can create confusion especially when reading texts translated into Spanish.

Between 10% and 15% of the western population is sterile or infertile.

Does age influence the possibility of becoming pregnant?

According to the SEF (Spanish Fertility Society), 25% of couples get a pregnancy in the first month of having regular and unprotected sex; 85% after 1 year, and 90% after 2 years.

For this reason, it is recommended to perform the basic study of sterility after 1 year of seeking pregnancy without success. Given that the passage of time has a negative impact on a woman's fertility, if she was older than 35 years old, the couple should go after 6 months.

The society of the well-being has caused that the age of the woman when forming stable pair increases, which has consequences in its future fertility. Currently in Spain, the average age of the woman in the first birth is 31 years. Sterility at 30 years is 6 times higher than at 20 and again at 40 years. The fertility of men decreases progressively after 50 years, although alterations in the parameters of the sonogram can be observed from the 25 but with much less importance than in women.

I hope this book was able to help you to understand what positive parenting is and I also hope that you will apply it in your life with your children.

The next step is to practice each and everything that is mentioned in this book.

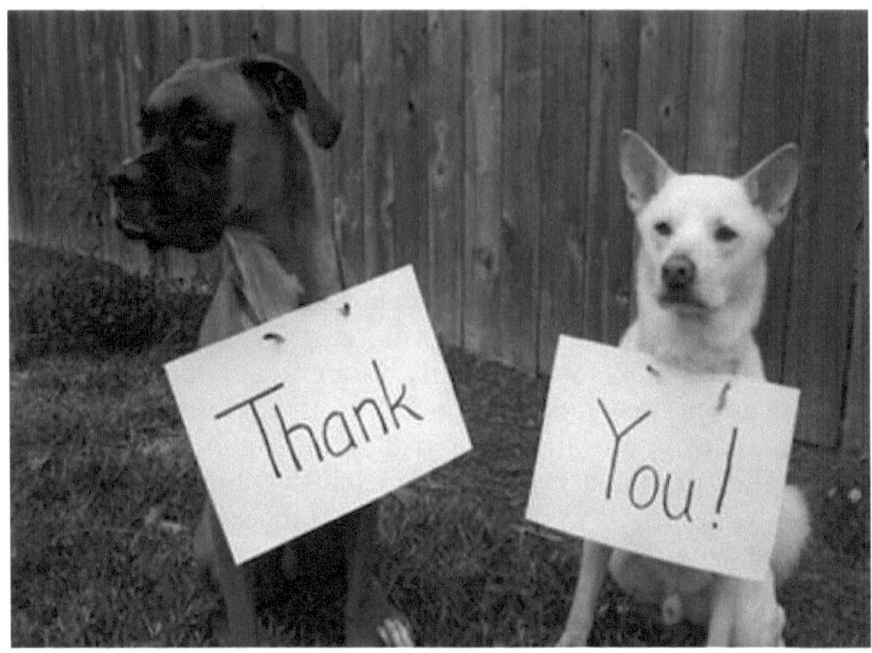

Finally, if you enjoyed this book, then I'd like to ask you for a favor, would you be kind enough to leave a review for this book on Amazon? It'd be greatly appreciated!

Thank you and good luck!

www.ingramcontent.com/pod-product-compliance
Lightning Source LLC
Chambersburg PA
CBHW051407280526
45784CB00007B/3128